Contents

Thank you for buying this book and I hope that you will find it useful. If you will want to share your thoughts on this book, you can do so by leaving a review on the Amazon page, it helps me out a lot.

Introduction

Sleep apnea is a condition when you briefly stop breathing while you're sleeping, or the breaths that you take are shallow. The momentary breathing can last from a couple of seconds and go on for a couple of minutes. These breathing disruptions can occur many times an hour, even more than 30 times within that 60-minute time period.

Later on, you would generally breathe once again. It might be accompanied by loud snoring or choking. This condition can hinder you from getting a good night's sleep. It causes you not to get as much sleep as you require. Sleep apnea induces you to be exhausted and drowsy throughout the day.

This condition is not one of those that are quickly diagnosed. Additionally, it is generally not discovered throughout a routine exam with your doctor. Since it occurs while you are sleeping, you most likely would not know that you had it unless somebody notices an uncommon pattern in your sleeping.

You might find out that you have sleep apnea if someone notices that as you are sleeping. Even then, they most likely will not understand that you might have sleep apnea.

Countless grownups are struggling with sleep apnea and do not understand it. Most of them are obese or overweight. Men struggle with this condition more than ladies. The older an individual is, the more likely they can inherit this condition. With ladies, they can develop sleep apnea in the post-menopausal phase of their life.

Minority groups, like African-Americans, Hispanics and Pacific Islanders develop sleep apnea more than other ethnic groups. It can additionally be inherited from members of the family. If you have little air passages in your throat, mouth or nose, you are more prone to having this condition.

Young kids that have larger than regular tonsil tissues can additionally establish sleep apnea. You can additionally be at risk for sleep apnea if you:

- Smoke.

- Have hypertension.

- Potential for having a stroke.

- Heart Failure

Chapter 1: Classifications Of Sleep Apnea

There are 3 kinds of sleep apnea, yet just 2 are discussed the most. There is obstructive sleep apnea, which is the most frequent type for this condition. With obstructive sleep apnea, your throat muscles collapse as you're sleeping.

The other kind of sleep apnea is referred to as central sleep apnea. This type occurs when your breathing muscles do not get the appropriate signals. The third one, which many people do not experience, is called complex or mixed sleep apnea. This kind is a mix of both conditions.

Obstructive Sleep Apnea

Obstructive sleep apnea, or OSA, obstructs the air passage in your throat. Some other things that occur with this kind of sleep disorder are:

- As you're sleeping, the throat muscles collapse inward as you're breathing.

- Air is going to pass through the upper airway. This consists of the nose, mouth and throat areas.

- As the muscles get broader, they obstruct the collapse in order for the airway to stay open.

- You are going to have less oxygen in your blood. This induces your lungs to take in air from the outside.

- Apnea occurs when the back throat tissues are momentarily obstructed. You stop breathing, and if you wake up, you might need to gasp for breath.

- Even when you do gasp for air or make snorting sounds, you might not always get up.

In case you experience 5 or more apnea episodes per hour, it is considered to be part of obstructive sleep apnea.

Central Sleep Apnea

Central sleep apnea is not as frequent as obstructive sleep apnea. This kind of sleep apnea begins in the brain. The brain will not send a signal to the airway muscles so that they can breathe.

The level of oxygen declines, and you are going to most likely wake up. With this kind of sleep apnea, individuals typically remember waking up. If you have heart disease or cardiac arrest, then you are experiencing central sleep apnea.

Complex or Mixed Apnea

As pointed out previously, this is the mix of obstructive and central sleep apnea. With this kind of sleep apnea, you are going to deal with obstructive sleep apnea, or OSA. In addition to that, with good pressure from the airway, you are going to have continual central sleep apnea.

If you are utilizing CPAP (Continuous Positive Airway Pressure), the central sleep apnea is going to be acknowledged. This occurs after the obstruction has actually been cleared.

Chapter 2: Symptoms and Signs

The most apparent symptom of sleep apnea is snoring that is loud and constant. You might pause while you are snoring. You might additionally choke or gasp after you have paused. Whenever you sleep on your back, the snoring gets louder. In case you sleep on your side, the snoring might not be as loud.

You might or might not snore every night. Ultimately, the snoring might increase, and it might get louder as you sleep.

Considering that you're sleeping while you're snoring or gasping, you might not know that you're having breathing problems. Others are going to see the indications before you and are going to let you know if it ends up being a pattern. Understand that just because you might be a chronic snorer, it does not indicate that you have sleep apnea.

If you are dealing with sleep throughout the day, that could be an indication that you have sleep apnea. If you're not engaged in any activity, you might wind up going to sleep really rapidly. If this occurs while you're at work or you're driving, the odds are higher that you might wind up in a work-related accident or an accident as you're driving.

There are other symptoms and signs that individuals might not connect with sleep apnea. They are:

- Headaches in the early morning

- Regular urination in the evening or night hours

- Moodiness or experiencing a change in your character

- Can't focus, concentrate or loss of memory

- Dry throat in the early morning as you get up

The muscles in your throat are utilized to keep the airway open to ensure that you can get air into your lungs. Nevertheless, when you're sleeping, your throat muscles are relaxed. This suggests that your airway can be obstructed, and air will not enter into your lungs.

With obstructive sleep apnea, you can additionally experience the following:

- If you have a small structure at the head and neck, the size of the airway might be tinier in your mouth and throat.

- The muscles in your throat and your tongue are more relaxed than they ought to be.

- Being obese or overweight, you will have extra soft fat tissue. This tissue can get thick in the windpipe wall. There is very little of an opening, and what is out there might not remain open.

- If you are an older grownup, the signals of your brain might not keep the muscles of your throat stiff like they ought to.

- With the obstructed air passages, you might wind up snoring loudly as you sleep.

Low oxygen levels cause you not to be capable of getting a good night's sleep. The muscles in the upper air passage get tight, and your windpipe is open. You have the ability to breathe ordinarily again until you begin snorting or choking.

Together with the frequent low levels of oxygen and fewer hours of sleep, your stress hormones are discharged. This can cause you to have hypertension, a stroke, cardiac arrest and irregular heartbeats. The stress hormones can additionally lead to you having a cardiac arrest.

If your condition is not dealt with, you might be at a higher risk of obesity and diabetes.

Chapter 3: Diagnosis Of Sleep Apnea

The manner in which doctors diagnose sleep apnea depends upon medical and family histories. They will additionally carry out a physical exam. They will study your signs. If they feel that the indications, signs and patterns fit this condition, then you are going to be referred for a sleep study.

Sleep studies are measurements that reveal your sleeping pattern. The outcomes demonstrate how much and how well you sleep. If you have any issues with your sleeping, the studies are going to reveal the results of that.

If you are referred for a sleep study, it is essential that you get one. The study can figure out if you have actually been diagnosed with a sleep disorder, like sleep apnea. Sleep apnea and other sleep disorders can boost your health risk for strokes, hypertension and cardiac arrest.

Physicians who are experienced in reading sleep studies can quickly detect sleep apnea and supply treatment so that you can sleep better during the night. The essential thing is to let your doctor know about any unfavorable sleeping habits you have experienced.

They would include tiredness and chronic drowsiness throughout the day. Additionally, advise your doctor if you have actually had trouble getting to sleep or getting up in the middle of the night and can't return to sleep.

You could be struggling with a sleep disorder that you are unaware of. Physicians experienced in sleep disorders are going to ask you about your sleep schedule. They are going to additionally ask your members of the family about any chronic snoring that they have actually handled.

Physicians who are experienced with sleep disorders are referred to as sleep specialists. They can quickly identify and supply the treatment for those who are experiencing issues sleeping.

In order to assist the specialists in identifying what's going on, you ought to establish and keep a sleep journal for no more than 2 weeks. This is the start of the sleep study. Here are some questions that you might see in a sleep journal:

- The time you went to sleep the night before

- The time you got up in the morning

- The number of hours you slept the night before

- The number of times you got up throughout the night

- How long did it take you to drop off to sleep the night before

- What medications you took the night before

- If you were you wide awake when you woke up in the morning

- If you were drowsy when you got up in the morning

- The number of drinks with caffeine you had throughout the day

- The number of beverages you had throughout the day

- The time when you drank the alcoholic drinks

- The number of naps you had

- The length of those naps

- If you were really drowsy throughout the day

- If you were a little tired throughout the day

- If you were relatively alert throughout the day

- If you were wide awake throughout the day

Your doctor might additionally inquire about the following:

- Snorting.

- Gasping.

- Headaches in the morning.

If the results of the journal point to:

- Regular naps.

- Waking up more than a couple of times throughout the night.

- Needing more than a half-hour to fall sleep.

- Continuously being drowsy in the daytime.

Physical Examinations To Check For Sleep Apnea.

Throughout the physical examination, your doctor will examine the areas of your throat, nose and mouth. They will be trying to find enlarged or extra tissues. For kids who are diagnosed with sleep apnea, they generally have enlarged tonsils. With them, it does not take much to provide a medical diagnosis aside from an examination and medical history.

For grownups, the doctors try to find an enlarged uvula, which is a piece of tissue that sits and hangs from the middle of the rear of your mouth. They additionally search for a soft palate, which remains in the back of your throat and is referred to as the roof of your mouth in that place.

How Family Members Can Aid To Identify Sleep Apnea.

Due to the fact that many people do not understand that they're struggling with sleep apnea, it is essential that there is somebody that can identify irregularities while you sleep. The individual does not know that their breathing can begin and stop at any time throughout the night. They additionally do not take into account when somebody tells them that they are chronic and loud snorer.

There are things that members of the family can do to assist:

- Letting a member of the family know that they have a chronic case of loud snoring.

- Telling them to consult their doctor.

- In case they are diagnosed with sleep apnea, advising them to follow the directions, consisting of any post-op, follow-up, and treatments.

- Being there for them emotionally. This could be a trying time for them, and they require all of the assistance that they can get.

Chapter 4: How To Diagnose Sleep Apnea With Sleep Studies

Sleep studies are generally carried out in a sleep center or a sleep laboratory. This might or might not be in a medical facility. If the study is performed in the sleep center, you might have an overnight stay. Nevertheless, this is not always engraved in stone.

The beneficial thing about sleep studies is that you will not endure any discomfort. The only thing that might impact you is skin irritation from the sensors. When the sensing units are removed from your skin, you will not deal with any more irritation.

Although the risks of sleep studies are marginal, these studies take some time (at least a couple of hours).

There are various tests for sleep studies. One of them is referred to as a polysomnogram or PSG test. This test is performed in a sleep center or sleep laboratory. More than likely, with this test, an overnight stay will be required.

You are going to have electrodes and monitors on your scalp, face, chest, limbs and fingers. As you are sleeping, the following things are going to be monitored:

- The motion of your eyes

- The activity in your brain

- The activity in your muscles

- The pace of your heart

- The tempo of your heart

- Blood pressure

- Air motion in and out of your lungs

- How much oxygen is in your blood

As you sleep, the staff on duty are going to utilize sensors to examine your as you sleep throughout the night. After the PSG is done, the sleep expert is going to go over the results with you. They are going to have the ability to identify whether you have sleep apnea and if it is serious or not. From the results, they are going to have the ability to chart a course of treatment.

A Multiple Sleep Latency Test or MSLT is utilized to identify how drowsy you are in the daytime. This test is generally carried out after a PSG. You will have devices put on your scalp for monitoring reasons.

With this test, you are going to need to take at least 5 naps, each lasting 20 minutes. This is supposed to be carried out every 2 hours throughout times when you would be alert. The testers are going to examine how long it is going to take you to go to sleep and how long you slept.

Those individuals who take less than 5 minutes to get to sleep are more likely prospects for a sleep disorder. When the screening is carried out, the sleep specialist is going to supply you with the results and talk to you about treatment options.

Where To Locate A Sleep Specialist

If you require help discovering a sleep specialist, there are a number of organizations that can help you with that, like:

- American Academy of Sleep Medicine (AASM)

- American Board of Sleep Medicine (ABSM)

- American Academy of Dental Sleep Medicine (AADSM)

These organizations are comprised of doctors, scientists and dentists that work with individuals impacted with this sleep disorder. They work to further the development of sleep medicine and sleep research.

The doctors and researchers that serve on the relevant boards are noted as "Board Certified" in the niche of sleep medicine. The ABSM keeps an updated listing of sleep specialists. They could be found by the state or by their name. The AADSM keeps an updated listing of dentists that focus on dealing with sleep apnea patients by utilizing oral devices.

Chapter 5: Kids With Sleep Apnea.

Kids who are diagnosed with sleep apnea could be hyperactive and aggressive. They can additionally suffer considerably in their studies. Often they might sleep in a different way than ordinary. They might additionally wet the bed. Throughout the daytime hours, a few of them are going to breathe through their mouth instead of breathing through their nose.

Snoring loudly, snorting, gasping for air and momentary stoppage in breathing all are indications of sleep apnea. Essentially, their symptoms and signs are parallel with what grownups have.

Even with this, doctors can not constantly spot this sleep disorder in kids. They figure that it's not a big deal due to the fact that most of them are hyperactive anyhow.

There are some things that you might do to discover if your kid, in fact, has sleep apnea:

- Talk to your kid's pediatrician and let them know what's happening.

- Talk to an ENT (ear, nose and throat) specialist.

- Talk to a pulmonologist (lung specialist) that specializes in kids.

- Psychiatrists, psychologists and other medical providers can additionally aid with a medical diagnosis.

If you have medical insurance, make certain to talk to them initially to see if you require referrals for particular medical providers.

If there is additional testing to be carried out, check to see if the doctors are board-certified to deal with kids with sleep apnea. Do not hesitate to inquire about their credentials. Besides, this is your kid's health that you're handling. With them, any medical diagnosis can need delicate care and consideration.

The doctor will additionally need to know if they are taking medications and if the kid is allergic to anything. Additionally, advise them of any problems with their habits and development. Along with that, supply them with information on their nighttime sleep patterns and if they take naps.

The kid might need to take a sleep study or polysomnogram (PSG) to identify the seriousness of their sleep apnea. There are other tests that are given to make a determination. They consist of:

- An electroencephalogram (EEG), which is utilized to assess the waves of the brain;

- An electrooculogram (EOG), which is utilized for chin and eye measurements;

- An electrocardiogram (EKG), which is utilized for tempo and heart rate measurements;

- Tests utilizing chest bands for breathing motion measurements;

- Tests utilizing more monitors for levels of oxygen and levels of co2 in the kid's blood.

Most of the sleep studies for kids call for an overnight stay. There are not a great deal of medical facilities that focus on sleep apnea for kids. Even with that, the ones that are utilized for grownups will use them to test kids too.

Check the facility to learn if they work with kids that might have this sleep disorder. Just like grownups, check different organizations and groups to locate a certified sleep specialist.

Additionally, similar to grownups, if sleep apnea goes without treatment in kids, they can additionally experience severe health problems down the road. Kids can additionally worsen with their behavioral patterns and academics in school if they are not dealt with in a timely manner. Do not take for granted

that they might simply be going through a tough time when it might very well
be sleep apnea.

Chapter 6: Treatments For Sleep Apnea

The function of dealing with sleep apnea (obstructive) is to enable the patient to be capable of breathing routinely as they sleep. The treatment additionally aids in getting relief from snoring loudly and being chronically drowsy throughout the day.

Treatment of sleep apnea additionally aids in decreasing medical issues, such as heart disease, diabetes, hypertension and other medical conditions.

Kinds of Treatments

There are various kinds of treatments to utilize for sleep apnea. Here are a few of the more typical ones:

- Lifestyle modifications

- CPAP.

- Mouthpiece or oral appliance.

- Surgery.

- Therapies.

With treatment, you can get more sleep and do away with being tired and drowsy throughout the daytime. Your general health is going to improve together with you being happier that you have the ability to get more sleep without being interrupted during the night.

It can additionally help the person sleeping next to you to get more sleep too. You will not be interrupting them by getting up at various times of the night, making snoring and gasping noises.

Chapter 7: Lifestyle Modifications.

In case you sleep on your back, you are subject to establishing sleep apnea. The way you set up yourself as you lie down on the bed can make or break you. It can determine the number of times you experience obstructive sleep apnea. It additionally determines how moderate or severe sleep apnea can impact you.

In some cases, it has to do with gravity. Gravity can cause your throat not to obtain ample air when you are resting on your back. Those who sleep on their backs can experience as much as 80 apneas per hour. They can do away with this problem by sleeping either on their left or right side. Nevertheless, if you are obese or overweight, this might not assist much.

You can make some lifestyle modifications in order to take care of obstructive sleep apnea and central sleep apnea:

- If you are obese or overweight, dropping weight can help. Weight loss can assist your throat to be less limiting. Eat more healthy vegetables and fruits. Be more physically active. If you are unsure how to set about losing weight, talk to your doctor.

- Leave the sleeping tablets and related medicines alone. Additionally, do not consume alcohol as a sedative to get you to sleep.

- The passageway of your nasal area must not be obstructed. If you have difficulty keeping them open, utilize a nasal spray or stick. You can additionally utilize decongestants, yet it's not for long-lasting usage.

- If you are used to sleeping on your back, that can pose an issue. Attempt sleeping on your side or your stomach. If you sleep on your back, your tongue and soft palate of your throat are going to sit on the back. This generates an obstruction of the throat's airway.

- Raise the head of your bed to boost your level of oxygen that you're ingesting.

- If you smoke cigarettes, you are going to need to quit as soon as possible.

Alternative medicine treatments, such as acupuncture, have been utilized to deal with sleep apnea, yet there is more research to be done. Because of this, do not utilize this technique as a means to get rid of this condition. Speak with your doctor prior to thinking about any alternative treatment for sleep apnea.

Chapter 8: Other Treatments For Sleep Apnea

If lifestyle modifications do not aid in treating your sleep apnea, then your case is more serious than what you initially believed. Here are some other treatments that might aid:

CPAP (Continuous Positive Airway Pressure).

CPAP (Continuous Positive Airway Pressure) is a technique where a machine generates air pressure. In order to get it, you need to put on a mask. The mask is positioned on your nose while you're sleeping.

When you are utilizing CPAP, you get more air pressure than you would if you were simply breathing in air from the outside. The air pressure with this machine assists in keeping the passageways of your upper airway open. This aids in preventing snoring and apnea.

Initially, not everybody that utilizes this machine will feel comfy with it. Due to the way it's made, it might not feel right in the beginning. Nevertheless, with modifications and making the straps fit appropriately, you will have the ability to get used to donning it.

Nevertheless, if the mask you have is not settling in, then you might need to discover another one. In addition to that, you can utilize a humidifier in addition to the CPAP for extra comfort.

There might be times when you have other issues. Nevertheless, do not stop utilizing it. Rather, check with your doctor to see what can be done and make extra corrections or adjustments. If you have actually put on weight, the settings for the air pressure need to be modified.

Possible Side Effects With CPAP

Throughout the very first couple of nights that you don this device, it can get on your nerves due to the fact that it is not immediately comfortable to wear. It makes you wish to stop the treatment for sleep apnea. Nevertheless, it would defeat the purpose. You can utilize the device with low air pressure at first.

The majority of people that utilize CPAP say that they experience side effects. The majority of them are managing the mask itself. You can pick a mask that provides comfort and stops it from leaking a great deal of air pressure.

Here are a few of the side effects that you might experience with the device:

- Irritated eyes.

- More air pressure than usual-- you can have a tough time breathing out when that takes place.

- Experiencing infections in the upper respiratory area if you do not keep the device tidy.

- Nose and throat irritation.

- Dry mouth.

- Sore mouth.

- Blockage in the nasal area.

- Nose sores from putting on the device too tight.

- The discomfort of the chest muscles

There are going to be other times when the CPAP will need to be calibrated. Your doctor or a sleep specialist can teach you how to do this. As soon as you discover how to do it, you will have the ability to save cash by not needing to make visits to see your doctor or specialist (unless absolutely required).

You can additionally get devices that are going to aid you to get more air in your throat. They are adjustable and made to fit your requirements in order to get more air flowing through your throat. The device calibrates the air pressure while you're sleeping. You do not need to press a button or utilize a dial to adjust it. The adjustment is made instantly as you sleep.

A mouthpiece or an oral appliance is an additional option if the CPAP does not work out for you. This device is utilized to keep your throat open to ensure that you can get air. It can assist those who are dealing with moderate sleep apnea.

Despite the fact that the CPAP is more helpful than the mouthpiece, the latter has actually been proven more convenient for some individuals to utilize while they're sleeping. It opens your throat by moving your lower jaw forward. Doing this can aid your snoring and treat moderate obstructive sleep apnea.

You can get a mouthpiece from a dental practitioner. It might take time to locate the ideal one that you can be comfy with. It is necessary that you talk to the dentist every 6 months after you begin using it.

After the first year of wearing, you can talk to the dentist once a year. You wish to ensure that it is still fitting right and working correctly. If you are feeling any pain, do not be reluctant to call the dentist for a possible adjustment.

Surgery

Surgery is another alternative to utilize in order to deal with sleep apnea. With the surgical procedure, excess tissue is extracted from your nose or your throat. This procedure is just carried out in a hospital.

Another alternative is to shrink or stiffen the extra tissue or the lower jaw could be reset. When the tissue is being shrunk or stiffened, the treatment is typically carried out in a doctor's office or in a hospital.

If the shrinking treatment is carried out, you might need to get some shots in the tissue area. If the excess tissue has to be shrunk more, you might require other treatments besides the shots. Additionally, the stiffening process consists of the doctor creating a little cut in the excess tissue and putting a little piece of plastic that is stiff.

Throughout the pre-surgery, you are going to be administered some medicine that is to make you go to sleep. So, throughout the surgery, you will be out and not feel anything up until you awaken. When the surgery is carried out in the hospital, you might experience pain in your throat lasting between 7 days and 14 days.

Here are some surgical options to deal with sleep apnea and aid you to rest better:

- UPPP (Uvulopalatopharyngoplasty) This is a treatment where tissue is extracted from the back of your mouth. The tissue is additionally taken out from the top part of your throat. In addition to getting rid of tissue, your tonsils and adenoids are additionally taken out.

With this surgery, your snoring might stop; nevertheless, considering that there is still tissue further down in your throat, it is not likely that it is going to treat or cure your sleep apnea. With the tissue staying there, your airway is closed. With UPPP surgical treatment, you will need to go to a hospital to have the surgery.

With this surgical treatment, you will experience a great deal of pain. You will be recovering for numerous weeks. This surgery is just carried out on individuals who are experiencing severe obstructive sleep apnea. Even then, there are just some who undergo this treatment.

This is not one of those surgeries where you can get up, and it's back to business as usual. If you have the ability to have the UPPP surgery, you might run the risk of having some complications, including:

- The soft palate and throat muscles might not work correctly.

- Your throat might get infected if no antibiotics are provided before the surgical treatment.

- You might have issues swallowing.

- You might experience fluids coming up through your mouth or your nose.

- You might not have the ability to smell.

It is not guaranteed that surgery will make you feel better. You might still have a reoccurrence of sleep apnea episodes. Even utilizing CPAP will not be as helpful after the surgery. There are some oral surgeries that can be carried out:

- A tracheostomy-- this surgery is carried out if previous treatments did not assist you. It is additionally utilized if your sleep apnea is serious to the point where it's a matter of life or death.

From an opening in your neck, a tube made from metal or plastic is put in and utilized for you to breathe from. The opening remains covered in the daytime and exposed during the night. You need air to go in and out of your lungs as you sleep.

- Maxillomandibular advancement-- This surgery is utilized to prevent blockage of your throat by making the space bigger where your tongue and soft palate are located.

The upper and lower part of your jaw is moved toward the front. This is how the enlargement is produced. This procedure is complicated, and an oral surgeon and orthodontist might need to do it together.

Surgeons utilize lasers to do away with unneeded tissues in the back of your throat. They can additionally utilize radiofrequency energy. Both of these procedures are great to utilize for dealing with snoring. Although they can be utilized to alleviate snoring, they must not be utilized to deal with obstructive sleep apnea.

There are more procedures that are utilized to alleviate snoring. A few of them can aid with dealing with sleep apnea. Nevertheless, the procedures are not cures for this sleep condition.

They consist of:

- Removing enlarged tonsils or adenoids

- Nasal surgery-- polyps are taken out, or a partition placed in between your nostrils is straightened out.

Extra surgical procedures that are utilized might deal with irregularities on your face. There are additionally surgical procedures that deal with extra blockages. Both of these can cause you to have sleep apnea. The procedures could be carried out together or solo.

Other surgeries include:

- Plastic surgery on the chin

- Tongue advancement-- this procedure entails a cut at the crossway of the jawbone and the tongue.

- Hyoid surgery-- the bone beneath the chin that can move is moved toward the front. As it moves, the muscle of the tongue moves along with it.

Having surgery to deal with apnea is not a guarantee. It depends upon what type of surgery it is and the particulars of the sleep apnea.

For central and complex sleep apnea, various therapies could be utilized. A few of them include:

- CPAP (Continuous Positive Airway Pressure).

- Medical treatments for neuromuscular problems.

- BiPAP (Bilevel Positive Airway Pressure)-- This is when greater pressure is utilized for breathing in. When you breathe out, the air pressure gets lower. This aids in reinforcing your breathing pattern if you have central sleep apnea. The device could be set to automatic mode if it spots that you have not breathed into it after a couple of seconds.

- ASV (Adaptive servo-ventilation)-- This is a new airflow device that gets a taste of how you breathe ordinarily. It keeps your breathing pattern information in a computer.

As long as you're sleeping, the ASV works to keep your breathing pattern at an ordinary rate and to get rid of any breathing pauses. In case you have central sleep apnea, this technique might work better for you than CPAP.

Sleep Apnea Pillows

There are some individuals who do get the advised quantity of sleep, yet they still get up tired. This can be linked to their snoring. Snoring is a really serious medical concern. To deal with that, sleep apnea pillows could be utilized.

Sleep apnea pillows have actually been known to deal with sleep apnea in some individuals. Before you attempt one, you need to understand whether you are simply snoring or if the snoring is an outcome of sleep apnea (obstructive).

Sleep apnea pillows can aid the airway of your throat to remain open. Due to the fact that sleep apnea causes your breathing to be uneven and disrupted, the pillow works to make your breathing regular again. The uneven and disrupted breathing typically occurs throughout the night when you are sleeping.

The special pillows are developed with panels of foam that are elevated, unlike a normal pillow. The elevation works to keep your head slanted. This aids to increase your breathing pattern to render it regular and undisturbed once again.

Sleep apnea pillows can be created to where they can be utilized in more than one sleeping position. They are flexible so that you can sleep in a manner in which is most comfy for you. They offer you with a great deal of assistance so that you can get a good night's sleep.

The sleep apnea pillow additionally assists in the following ways in regard to sleep apnea:

- Obstructed airways are opened-- this aids with snoring relief and sleep apnea

- Supplies comfort and assistance to ensure that you can obtain a good night's sleep

- Alleviates you from the fatigue that you experience due to your sleep apnea condition

- The pillow enables you to sleep like a newborn

There are individuals who are chronic snorers that have actually never utilized these kinds of pillows and do not wish to try them. They would rather get sleeping tablets and wind up getting dependent on them. Medication is not a great alternative to help you with your snoring or sleep apnea. Actually, medication is not advised since it has actually proven not to be helpful.

Chapter 9: Crucial Points About Sleep Apnea

Here are some essential points that you ought to understand about sleep apnea:

- Sleep apnea is a chronic condition in which your sleep is disrupted more than 3 nights weekly.

- Due to the fact that snoring is ordinary for some individuals, this sleep disorder can be easily be ignored.

- Obstructive sleep apnea is the most frequent of the 3 that are pointed out.

- Being chronically sleepy in the daytime can cause you to have a work-related mishap.

- If you are obese or overweight and struggling with sleep apnea, work on getting your weight down. When you do, do not put the pounds back on.

- A member of the family can determine something might be wrong when the individual is choking and gasping for air and not getting ample sleep.

- There are various ways to get treated for sleep apnea. Depending upon the intensity of your condition, the doctor and sleep specialist are going to work to get the most effective treatment for you.

- Individuals must not make fun of those who are struggling with sleep apnea. This is a really considerable sleep condition that needs to be treated with urgency.

- Kids that have behavioral issues and problems with academics are frequently ignored. These indications are typically not associated with sleep apnea.